Not Likely

Defeating Cancer & Stupidity

Version 8

ISBN: 9781688077614

Dedication

To my Family.

Contents

Forward

Names withheld for privacy concerns.

This book is a true story about my last six years of fighting cancer and fighting stupidity. What I found was something I may not have realized if the worse of, the worse had not happened.

I am alive today because of the "Eight Rules to a Successful Life" (see chapter 18).

If you don't give up, you will never lose.

In this game, if I give up, I die.

I found a healthcare system that is out of control and killing people.

First, my doctors said nothing was wrong with me for over a year. Then I was told, don't worry, we can fix it. At that point, my life's course was headed toward falling off a cliff.

I discovered that Cancer was not my biggest enemy in my fight to stay alive.
See the Appendix for helpful information for cancer patients and their families.

1: The Beginning

I am speaking on the phone, "The doctor scoped my throat. The doctor said he is sure it is cancer." My voice cracked at the word cancer.

My sister did not understand what I said, so I had to repeat my diagnosis. Repeating it felt like I was giving bad news to myself again.

After a few weeks of saying, "I have cancer," the phrase almost seemed boring.

People are very adaptable. Any situation will become part of your day. A few months later, I was talking about a decision a doctor asked me to make. I said, "All these life-and-death decisions are starting to get boring." The doctor laughed; I was serious.

I am a computer professional; I ran a software development company for twenty-five years and was a CFO for a quasi-government agency. I have enjoyed amateur Ballroom Dancing for thirty-seven years. I am well known in Southern California as a dancer. I struggle to dance in Southern California without someone recognizing me. Ballroom dancing is something I love.

If you don't know where you are going, you can't get there.

The above is one of my favorite sayings about businesses which I should have applied to my life. I never set a grand goal for my life. Getting rich is not a goal (it is a by-product).

If you don't give up, you will never lose.

Computer software can be complicated with large installations. Software analysis and finding bugs can drive you nuts. My most exceptional skill in software analysis was not my intelligence or knowledge base; I never gave up. I knew I would solve the problem, whatever it was, though I did not know how long it would take.

Giving up does happen in this computer field. The end-user will hear from the programmer, "you will just have to live with it," or "code is a little quirky," or "it is on our list." I never gave up on researching a bug.

Never giving up is crucial to my story.

What I learned from Chapter 1:

The most important part of chapter 1 is you need a plan (a goal). You can cruise through life with no plan and end up old and wondering what happened. Where did the time go?

Never give up is a phrase to use with having a plan. It is easier never to give up if you have a goal.

2: The Art of Medicine

The term "practicing the art of medicine" refers to the practice of medical care as a profession in which medical knowledge and skills are applied in a compassionate, ethical, and effective way. It involves using scientific knowledge, technical skills, and the ability to listen and communicate with patients, make sound judgments and decisions, and adapt to changing situations.

The art of medicine involves the ability to identify and address patients' physical, emotional, and social needs and work with them to develop a treatment plan that meets their individual needs and goals. It requires the ability to think critically, problem-solve, and use a range of tools and resources, including medications, therapies, and diagnostic tests, to diagnose and treat illness.

Practicing the art of medicine involves a commitment to ongoing learning and professional development and staying current with advances in medical knowledge and techniques. It also consists of a commitment to ethical principles and upholding the highest professional conduct standards.

Dancing, I meet many different types of people from all over the world, from the good to the bad.

One of the good people was from Italy, a nurse, and her husband was a doctor. I found most nurses are seriously interested in other people's situations. She was no different; she was from the best of the best.

I do not usually teach people to dance. I prefer to fly across the dance floor with a partner that does not inhibit my dancing. I taught her how to waltz. She always remembered the lessons and that I was the one that helped her get started in ballroom dancing.

Years before I became seriously ill, I had a minor problem. I told her about it, and her husband showed up the next week to talk to me. He knew how to dance but did not like it as much as other things he wanted to do.

The Art of practicing medicine

At that time, she said, "It is called: "The Art of practicing medicine" for a reason." A doctor gave me a non-definitive diagnosis (they were unsure what the problem was). I'm not sure why I remembered what she said, but it helps explain what has happened to me recently (the last six years).

At one dance, she told me she had liver cancer, and the time she had left had passed two years ago.

I have not seen her for several years. I prefer to think she is still doing good wherever she goes.

For this journey, it is essential to realize that medicine is an art form, not a science. One doctor may tell you one thing, another doctor something completely different. Or several doctors may say to you the same thing.

One might think if many doctors are telling you the same thing, it must be correct. Not necessarily; they might just read your chart entries from the other doctor(s) and say that it makes sense.

If the doctors disagree, this might tell you something, or it may not. [Sorry, I am starting to sound like a doctor.] One of the doctors may have the correct answer, but how do you tell which is right?

One reason for the group diagnosis problem is most doctors are pushed to see at least a certain number of patients per hour in most healthcare establishments. They read a diagnosis on a patient's chart; they are most likely to agree with it or suggest minor changes.

One minor possibility is the doctor reviewing your chart does not like the other doctor; therefore, that doctor will come up with a completely different diagnosis. Doctors are human and have human emotions.

What can you do? Research. Start with friends and family, and discover if they were exposed to your symptoms or illness. Next, go to the internet. The internet is full of information, but not all are correct. Start with federal government websites (such as FDA.gov); the sites will end with ".gov." Some states may have additional information for you. I next go to the website WebMD.com (I have no association with them). WebMD has understandable information on diseases and drugs. Lastly, find online user groups. These are not usually professional medical people but may have additional ideas or options. Do not be suckered in by the vitamin pushers. Your doctor can run a blood test to see if you are malnourished.

How do I search the internet? I use DuckDuckGo.com (I have no association with them), not Google.com. DuckDuckGo does not give your search information to advertisers. A little privacy is always nice to enjoy.

You may want to research your doctor, but I have never had what I would call adequate information. There are several websites offering reviews of doctors. I have never found a website with a negative review for a doctor I researched (hard to believe, considering the care I received). If your doctor has lawsuits filed against them, you might be able to find them online. Type your doctor's name into a search engine, then start reading.

Your healthcare provider's website might give you general information about their doctors. You might be able to see what schools the doctor went to and what board specialties the doctor may possess.

You make your decision about what you want. You are in charge.

If you do not feel equipped to make such a decision, let your spouse, family, or close friend help you, or lastly, let your doctor decide on what to do. Never ignore it; if the doctor says the condition is serious, believe the doctor.

What I learned from Chapter 2:

Medicine is not an exact science. A doctor can tell you what usually the problem is from your symptoms. Unfortunately, that may not be what is wrong with you. Please research and ask for a second opinion; your life may depend on it.

Cherish the good people as you travel through life. Try to be a little more like their best attributes. Cherishing the good will make you a better person and make your life fuller.

3: Something is Wrong

I have never had a problem swallowing pills. I could take aspirin without a glass of water.

I struggled to swallow a single pill with a full glass of water. At the time, I thought my problem was not serious. My doctors did not seem concerned. The doctors prescribed this little test here and there, this drug and that drug. Ever so slightly, my frustration grew and grew.

Recently, a doctor who knew my history (of the past six years) told me that doctors also become very frustrated when they cannot find the cause of the problem.

Over a year passed, and I began having more problems and feeling bad all of the time. The many diagnoses and the drugs prescribed did not change what was happening. I got the feeling from my physicians that they might think I am a hypochondriac.

If you are not feeling well, the doctor is not helping you feel better. Find a new doctor.

Jump forward to now. In discussion with one of my many doctors (using the plural of doctor is not me bragging, but complaining), he described how a patient died. The patient had kept complaining about head pain. The doctors kept saying the cause of his headaches was his use of marijuana. He died shortly after the correct diagnosis when they discovered what was wrong (brain tumor).

One beautiful California morning, I was coughing up blood for a half hour. After I stopped coughing up blood, I went to the emergency room of my healthcare provider, which is half an hour away.

I showed the ER (emergency room) my medical card. I told them I'd been coughing up blood for half an hour. They immediately take me to an isolation room for examination. A doctor and two nurses stood around me, waiting for me to cough up blood. They are bound up in isolation clothing which they disposed of and put on new when they leave and come back into the isolation room.

In walks a woman in a business suit and clipboard, leaving the door open; she announces that I did not show my photo ID when I came into the ER. The doctor and two nurses took a giant step backward away from me. One of the nurses gave me the plastic bag with my clothes. I show the woman my driver's license. She left, closing the door. To me, this was an unbelievable attitude from my healthcare provider. It would not get better.

My body refused to cough up more blood. The doctor ordered a chest x-ray and sent me home. I left the ER with the feeling that they did not believe that I had been coughing up blood, but they would get their money (what seems to be most important to them).

In my family, I have a pretty good network of healthcare professionals. My sister is a nurse, my sister-in-law is a nurse, my sister's sister-in-law is a nurse, and my sister's good friend is a doctor. My family's feedback from my visit to the ER was not positive — frustration reigns.

If you don't give up, you will never lose.

The ER x-ray showed a "shadow" on my lungs; the doctors said, "it could be something" or "it could be nothing." My Frustration was at an unbelievable level. Semantically null statements frustrate me.

I do not know how to read x-rays; everything looks like a shadow.

A flurry of other scans happened, showing what might lead to a different type of scan. They threw in a stomach biopsy. This test leads my primary care doctor to say, "We have scanned every inch of your body; there is no cancer." I had never mentioned the word 'cancer" to him. He mentioned it several times, saying, "no cancer."

Months later, a doctor would re-examine the scans and find something horrible. All they had to do was look at the scan in the correct area of the scan.

What I learned from Chapter 3:

Suppose you know that something is seriously wrong. If the doctors tell you, you are fine. Please do not believe them; keep after them until you are satisfied.

You are in charge. It is your life; you are the customer; make the medical staff respect you and your condition.

4: Dumb and Dumber – not the movie

The doctors settled on a diagnosis of 'nervous throat and dry sinus.' The doctors never saw me cough up blood.

I got a prescription for my nervous throat. My primary care doctor prescribed a Neti pot. A device that you use to pour a saline solution up your nose to clean out your sinuses. Not fun, but painful.

One morning I coughed up some blood. I wiped up the blood this time and put it in a plastic bag. My primary doctor was not in, but another doctor was available to see me. My thought was great. I will get a second opinion from a different primary care doctor. She only glanced at the plastic bag and said the sample I brought was useless. She looks up my nose. She tells me I am not using the Neti pot enough to use it more often.

About a week later, I coughed up some more blood. I again brought a sample of the blood. A third primary care doctor was available to see me. She carefully looks at the blood sample and then looks up at my nose. She tells me that either I'm using the Neti pot not enough or I'm using it too much.

The word stupid is used way too much in our society, so that I will use the word dumb. This advice is one of the dumbest pieces of advice I have ever received from a medical doctor. It is like saying, "you should have the surgery, or you should not have the surgery," or "it is critical you take this medication, or you mustn't take it." These are semantically null diagnoses. They say nothing.

I went home and threw out the Neti pot.

Over the previous few months, my primary doctor kept mentioning the "C" word, though I never said it.

I was feeling bad, horrible; I was dying before their eyes. I met up with my two sisters, niece, and great-niece. My sister (the nurse) said I looked horrible and I needed to take control of my treatment. (This advice saved my life)

I went in to see my main doctor (primary care physician). I made my second request to see an ENT (Ears, Nose, Throat doctor). My doctor said the same thing as before, "We have scanned every inch of your body, and there is no cancer. You can see an ENT, but it is not necessary." Again, I never mentioned the word cancer.

This time I insisted.   [Note life-saving event, almost]

Lesson: You are in charge if you think it might help insist.

What I learned from Chapter 4:

You are in charge; if you think it might help, insist on tests, get a new doctor, whatever it takes; your life depends on it. Be the most annoying person possible. The squeaky wheel gets the grease.

5: The Correct Diagnosis

I was finally in an ENT (Ears, Nose, Throat) doctor's office. ENT's are now called Face Neck Surgeons. Why was I so insistent on seeing an ENT? No one had looked at my neck. The doctors went from the lungs to the stomach and the sinus. The doctor doing the stomach biopsy did not pause a second to see how the throat looked. All of the doctors completely skipped over the throat. The scans included the throat, but the large cancer mass was not "noticed."

I told the ENT most of what happened over the previous 15 or so months. He examined me for **two minutes**. He said, "I know what is wrong; let me get a scope." It took him longer to find an endoscope than to reach his diagnosis.

An endoscope is a long narrow tube; with a camera inside. It is made to go inside your body. The doctor uses it to see what your body looks like inside. Some have video screens so the patient can see and allows screen recording. Other endoscopes have no video; only the doctor can see what is inside you.

I hate being right when it means I will die (die here is not an overstatement).

My ENT rolled in an endoscope with a video monitor.

"I'm sure it is cancer."

My ENT said, "See that? I'm sure it's cancer." I looked at the video screen as the cable traveled down my neck, it looked like cancer to me, and I had no idea what cancer should look like. I knew it was cancer. I knew I was in big trouble.

My ENT pointed out the cut cancer made in my throat. This is why I was coughing up blood.

I tell my family I have cancer. They are generally shocked but not completely surprised.

The next step is surgery to do a biopsy. A couple of weeks go by, waiting for the operation. It amazed me that they did not seem in a hurry. Cancer grows, destroys, and grows some more, destroys, etc. It does not take a holiday.

Several days after the biopsy, the surgeon seems to do an overelaborate setup for my visit to get the results. A nurse brought a box of tissues and placed it on a table next to me.

The result is cancer. I already knew that for weeks. I wonder how often they will tell me it is cancer before they start treating me.

After the biopsy, they scheduled a very long wait for an MRI (Magnetic Resonance Imaging). Again, I'm thinking about what is wrong with these people. I called a different hospital and asked how long it would take to get an MRI; they said I could come in tomorrow ($1,800). Lack of funds means I have to wait. This other hospital does not know I have cancer, but they could scan me immediately. I get a slightly shorter date (a few days) from my healthcare provider by agreeing to go to a different hospital in their healthcare network.

I now have a video of my throat showing cancer, a biopsy, and an MRI showing everywhere the tumors are located. Time from the initial diagnosis to getting treatment is turning into months.

I am sent to a different ENT. I don't know why. He asked if I wanted a 'doctor's analysis' (unsure of the exact term he used). I said, "Yes if it will get me treated." The analysis involved a bunch of interns who knew almost nothing looking at my throat—a training session for doctors (I was not told this would be a training session). After a long trip to northern Los Angeles, it is time to get treatment. Wrong!

They needed to have my teeth x-rayed. The teeth x-rays were necessary because radiation destroys everything it hits. Radiation therapy could have disastrous effects if a hole in a tooth (cavity) exists.

They were going to give me chemo (chemotherapy) & radiation treatment. Why? Surgically removing the cancer was not possible. It is now too large, more than a year and a half after the first signs of cancer presented itself.

Since my healthcare provider does not have a dentist on staff, they sent me to a university hospital for a dental exam. The hospital is rated as the fourth-best cancer institute in the world. I expected a department with leading-edge technology. Wrong, think 1950s technology.

OK, now get treatment? Nope. I was put on a waiting list to get chemo & radiation treatment.

Never give up.

What I learned from Chapter 5:

Never, never, never give up. If I had given up, I would be dead.

Make them do what you know has to be done. You will be healthier for it.

6: Cut it Out

Being a man of action, my first response to the cancer was, "cut it out, cut it out, cut it out."

"Go ahead and reach down my throat and yank it out," I told my surgeon, only half-joking. The surgeon did a biopsy surgery (my first biopsy surgery; this was before treatment). They put me entirely out where I stopped breathing, shoved a breathing hose down my throat to give me oxygen, cut biopsies, and sealed the cuts made by cancer-causing me to cough up blood.

After surgery, I needed the potent painkiller they gave me. I'm not a big fan of pain relievers, but this was necessary. The day after the surgery, I watched my clock to see when I could take the next dose of painkiller.

This surgery was the first of three biopsies surgeries. A different surgeon would perform the subsequent two surgeries. I do not know why I did not keep the same surgeon.

The cuts in my throat made by cancer were just an inch or two down from my throat opening. The ER doctors or a very long list of other doctors could have seen it if they had looked.

After my cancer diagnosis, doctors told me, "Don't worry; this is a good type of cancer."

I have been told the best way to deal with serious wrongs that happened in the past is to "Just let it go; it's in the past." I'm dying because of gross incompetence by multiple doctors and their healthcare management. I counted eight doctors in a row with a different diagnoses. "Get real 'philosophy types,' letting go is sometimes not an option or a good option." Anger can keep us aware of things, places, or people that harm us.

Anger can be a good thing

I noticed that I used anger at my healthcare provider to divert my mind from the fact that I might be dying. I was much angrier than being concerned about my coming death. My family mentioned that they thought I was worried about dying more than once. What they read as concern on my face was just physical pain.

Ronald Reagan's advice is critical when he said multiple times about Soviet treaties, "Trust but verify." Is your life at stake? Trust your doctor but make sure the doctor proves it repeatedly. I mean everything, not just one drug, the diagnosis, the treatment, everything.

What I learned from Chapter 6:

If it takes anger to get it done, use anger, but keep it in control. You need these people to cure you.

7: Radiation Therapy

Radiation therapy, or radiotherapy, is a cancer treatment that uses high-energy radiation to kill cancer cells or shrink tumors.

A machine directs a radiation beam at the cancer cells or tumor during radiation therapy. The high-energy radiation damages the DNA in the cancer cells, which can prevent the cells from growing and dividing. This can help shrink the tumor or kill the cancer cells.

Radiation therapy is usually given as a course of treatment over several weeks, and it is usually given five days a week. The length of treatment depends on the type and stage of the cancer being treated.

Radiation therapy can be used to cure cancer, control cancer, help alleviate symptoms, or to slow the progression of cancer. It is often combined with other cancer treatments, such as chemotherapy or surgery.

Radiation therapy can cause side effects, such as skin irritation, fatigue, and nausea. These side effects usually go away after treatment is completed.

Before starting treatment, my sister asked me how I felt about going in for radiation treatment. I said, "I will endure two months of horror, then I will be cured, and I will go on with my life." I cannot answer why I still trusted my healthcare provider to cure me.

The Mask.

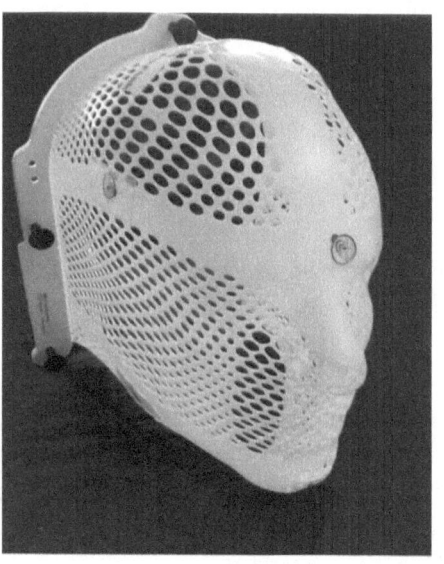

The mask was used to bolt my head down while I received radiation treatment (See picture of the radiation machine at the end of this chapter). My head was not on the table. I was clammed down to an attachment they used at the end of the table. The attachment felt like a wooden dowel with a towel wrapped around it. A little more than a month into treatment, the back of my head was incredibly sore. Each daily session was uncomfortable. I did not pay much attention to this pain since every cell in my body was screaming at me. I ignored my cells (they are whiny little bastards).

A couple of reasons it took so long to start my therapy, they needed to do the calculation for the radiation treatment angles, and they needed to make the mask.

To make the mask, they had me lay on the radiation bed. They bring over a crisscross hatched plastic, holding it like a hot potato. They drop the plastic on my face (it is scorching); the technicians take a spray bottle with water to wet it down so it will cool faster. I wonder why they did not wet my face before dropping the hot plastic on it.

Five days a week, I would see the machine below. They would check me outside the room and again inside it to ensure they had the correct person and radiation treatment. The door to the radiation room looked like a door to a bank vault.

The check-in and bolt-my-head-down process took longer than the actual radiation treatment, except for one day.

This radiation machine is also an x-ray machine. Once a week, the technicians would x-ray my head and neck to ensure I was positioned correctly on the radiation bed. After the x-ray, they would usually come in and shove me in one direction or another, a few times, while my head was bolted down (I felt like a piece of meat that they shoved around the meat counter).

After a few weeks, I was intimate with what the radiation machine made sounds and how it moved around me. It made a bee-like sound when it was shooting me with radiation.

One day, it sounded like trouble. It would start the buzzing, then stop, then start again. It stopped; every light in the place clicked on; I had never seen it so bright in this room.

A technician came into the room say that there was a problem with the machine. She asked, was there something she could do for me. I asked that the mask be removed, the wooden dowel be replaced with something more comfortable, and to get my water.

She said, " Okay, not to move because you are up in the air. I knew the table went up some, but it was between five and six feet in the air, far higher than I thought. I lay five/six feet up in the air for a half-hour waiting for them to fix the problem.

They fixed the problem; they put the wooden dowel back, bolted me down, and shot me full of radiation. When leaving the room, I heard someone say, "I'm sorry." I immediately turn around, saying, "What?" The guy says, "Nothing." For a short moment, it seems someone took responsibility for their actions.

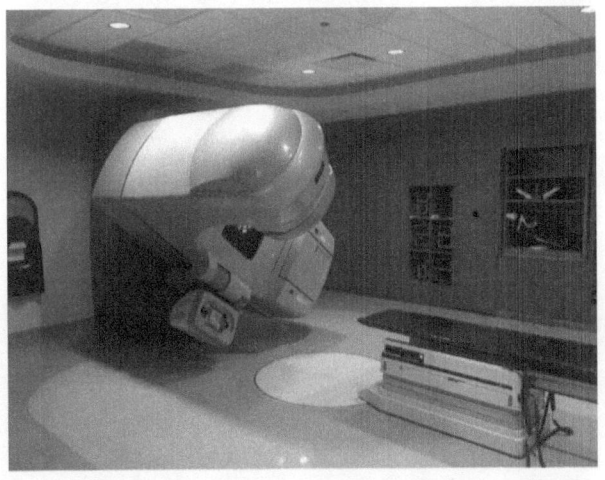

The machine.

The bed on the right is about ten feet long. At rest, the bed is about three feet high. The bed moves forward (toward the machine) and upward.

Two months of radiation treatments (70 grays, a lot) aged my face fifteen years. Every doctor that saw how much radiation I received would say, "that is a lot of radiation." One hundred grays of radiation is considered fatal. My healthcare provider said they would help restore my face (eliminate the years added).

Later they refused to help to restore my face. I was told they no longer do strictly cosmetic procedures anymore. They now only do medical procedures.

Now, anytime I go in for any radiation exam, I think about how much shorter my life will be. Radiation never leaves your body. Every dose of radiation shortens my life.

What I learned from Chapter 7:

Radiation is unpleasant but kills cancer and non-cancer cells if used correctly. If you are claustrophobic, you will need something to calm you down.

Check the doctor's credentials that are doing the calculations for your treatment.

8: Chemotherapy

Chemotherapy is a cancer treatment that uses drugs to kill cancer cells. Chemotherapy is usually given as a course of treatment over some time, and it may be delivered in different ways, such as orally (by mouth) or intravenously (through a vein).

Chemotherapy attacks rapidly dividing cells, which is more common in cancer cells than in normal cells. However, chemotherapy drugs also attack normal cells that divide quickly, such as those in the hair, stomach, and intestines; they can cause various side effects, including hair loss, nausea, and vomiting.

Chemotherapy is often combined with other cancer treatments, such as surgery or radiation therapy. It can be used to cure cancer, control cancer, help alleviate symptoms, or slow its progression.

Sitting in the hospital cafeteria with my sister, waiting to get my first chemo treatment, my head falls to the table, and I say, "There is no such thing as a 'good cancer.'"

I wouldn't say I like it when I'm right. In the past, I've had a girlfriend say to me, "Must you always be right?" I do not think that this situation is what she meant.

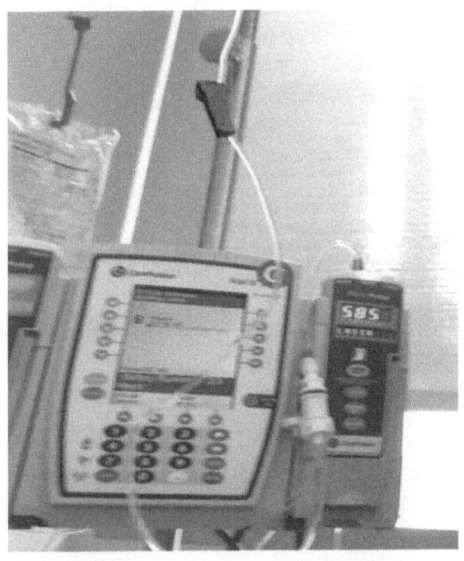

Pictured is the IV (intravenous) that delivered the chemo.

They make an annoying noise at the end to alert the nurses that the IV is complete. The nurses need a loud alarm since they continually run from patient to patient.

Chemo & radiation is a horrible journey. Taking the elevator on my first chemo treatment, we meet another couple. The couple was distraught. They were on their third type of chemo, which was not working. There are many types of chemotherapy treatments for different kinds of cancers. Cancer is not a single disease but several different types of illness.

The first chemo treatment gave me tinnitus (ringing in the ears). The ringing will never go away for the rest of my life. A doctor told me the ringing would go away if I went deaf. [for some doctors, there are not enough curse words]

Why I am not punching these doctors in the face, I do not know. I did not think to ask the doctor if I would go deaf.

In a recent discussion with my first ENT, he said I lost some hearing, but I am not out of the normal range of hearing.

I felt a little weaker whenever I walked out of the radiation room. Walking out of that room happened five times a week. I felt like the walking dead.

On Thursdays, I would go to the chemo department and then to radiation.

Switching to the second chemo drug gave me what the doctor warned me was acme. It did not look like acme to me. My face looked like something from a monster movie. Most of the acme would be gone in a few weeks.

What I learned from Chapter 8:

Chemo can be beneficial. Triple-check out the doctor who is in charge of your treatment. Ensure they tell you what you must be concerned about with your treatment. I was given a 40-page report and a video to watch. Snowing you with information is not acceptable. Insist on seeing your doctor and make him tell you what is likely.

9: You are Cured

When I met my Face Neck surgeon (my 2nd ENT doctor), I described the more than a year-long journey to meet him.

He said, unfortunately, it is not the first time he has heard a story like mine, where they found nothing because they were looking in the wrong place.

I liked his honesty.

After completing the chemo & radiation, I was told it would take months before they could scan me since the radiation had destroyed so much tissue that nothing would be distinguishable.

I did not feel right for those months.

My radiologist and 2nd ENT alternated scoping me. The radiologist would scope me for one month; the 2nd ENT would scope me the following month. This scoping continued past the PET scan. The scopes are painful, but humans can get used to almost anything.

I was concerned about how useful scoping was as a diagnostic tool; I complained that it looked on the outside of my inside. The camera saw my throat but nothing inside the tissue.

Unfortunately, I was correct about it being an ineffective diagnostic tool.

What I learned from Chapter 9:

Just because you like the doctor's personality does not mean they are the correct doctor for you. Write down a list of questions for the doctor. Make sure the doctor answers them to where you understand the answer.

Check at the end of this book for a list of questions. Add to that list any of your concerns.

10: Sell my Condo

Just because someone says something with authority does not mean they are correct for your situation.

I wanted to sell my condo in Long Beach. It was December; I was still undergoing chemo & radiation treatment. My agent told me December was a horrible time to sell my place. She wanted ninety days to sell it; I gave her thirty days.

I was living in my brother's place in Laguna Beach. It was less than four weeks to the end of my treatment. To get my condo ready for sale, I would drive from Laguna Beach to Anaheim to get my treatment. Then I would drive from Anaheim to Long Beach to move stuff and finish work on my condo. Then drive to my temporary home in Laguna Beach. Each segment of the trip was about a half-hour. How was I able to do this? Everything hurt, whether lying down watching TV or working in my place. I might as well be productive.

I was tolerating the treatment well. This does not mean the treatment was working well, just that I was functional (able to move independently), not throwing up, hair not falling out, etc. I felt like hell, like every cell in my body was exploding. Something similar to a horrible hangover that never went away twenty-four hours a day, seven days a week for months.

If you don't give up, you will never lose.

My condo sold in two days. My agent was amazed. About ten days later, I was offered another fifteen thousand, but I could not take it since I had already accepted the previous offer. I learned a lesson that cost me a bit of money. "Take a deep breath before accepting an offer."

Just because someone is excellent at their job does not mean they are always right.

My agent is excellent at her job. I have made several purchases with her. Even if a person is excellent at their job does not mean that they are always right.

I was still feeling like hell but with some money. I had to move all my stuff out of the condo and into storage. Done with my treatment, I had to find a new home.

I settled on a place less than ten minutes from the hospital (in Los Angeles County) where my adventure started. Anaheim and Laguna Beach are in Orange County. I selected my new place because I wanted to be close to a hospital and a dance studio I often visit.

I am moving into my new place. I do not feel well though the doctors do not think anything is wrong with me (Sound Familiar?). My new home needs a lot of work, both outside and inside.

I buy some new furniture but have no energy to change my new home significantly.

My new place was supposed to be a fresh start for me. Instead, I felt like hell.

What I learned from Chapter 10:

No matter how good a professional (doctor, real estate agent, etc.), they can make mistakes. Trust but Verify everything; it could mean your life.

11: My Family

Though I tolerated treatment well, my family did a better job of tolerating me. I cannot fathom how I would have gotten through this process without them being there for me.

I have a brother and two sisters, the big sister, is a retired nurse. My brother donated his condo and later money to get a second opinion.

I moved to my brother's vacation condo, which was much bigger than mine, so my sisters could move in with me.

They divided me up; my younger sister would start with me, then my older sister would come in for the latter part of treatment, where a professional nurse may be needed. Things that a professional should be watching over, like a feeding tube, oxygen, etc. I did not look forward to the second half of my treatment.

I found out something significant to me. I hate the way my sisters drive.

A couple of weeks into being driven by my little sister, I started driving myself to the hospital daily, and my sister was the passenger.

When my big sister arrived from Austin, Texas, she used my car to drive me to the hospital. My little sister went home. When we pulled into the parking lot of the radiation center, she asked me if I wanted to drive home. I said, "Yes." She said something profound like "Men!"

I drove to the hospital from thereon. About three weeks before the end of the treatment, my big sister stopped going with me to the hospital. It felt bizarre being alone in the car. There was nothing for her to do at the hospital.

Mid-way through the radiation treatment, I was told to start using the painkillers every four hours (the pain level would increase significantly). I went home, took a dose, and watched my watch for four hours. I took another dose. A couple of hours later, I decided it was not doing anything for me. I stopped taking the painkillers except sometimes to help me go to sleep (it did not help much with sleep either). After completion of treatment, I told a doctor what I did, and he just about fell off his chair in amazement.

You are in charge.

Ten days before the end of the treatment, my big sister went home. She had things to do at home. At Laguna Beach, she was taking walks on the beach. I was capable of doing anything I needed.

My brother's place is a two-story condo; the bedrooms are downstairs, and the living room, kitchen, and dining room are upstairs.

The morning after my sister went home to Texas, I got out of bed and walked upstairs. The place was tranquil.

I have never felt so lonely in all of my life. Instead of a sister yelling at me to eat more or get up and move, there was silence.

I sat on the couch for a while. All the cells in my body were yelling at me to please stop this madness.

Never give up.

I got up, got ready for the hospital, and drove.

Family is very important.

What I learned from Chapter 11:

There is one absolute constant in this universe. Your family is your family. Your family or close friends will want to help you but may not know what to do for you. Help them help you.

12: Surgery & Surgery

About four months after the completion of the chemo & radiation, a PET scan showed a "shadow." But it was "probably nothing." An endoscope showed something weird (weird is my word; the white dot is what they saw) toward the bottom of my throat.

I had classified Endoscopes as very uncomfortable. After the pain of chemo & radiation treatments, it now seems just uncomfortable.

My 2nd ENT did not think anything was wrong with me. He did not think I needed another biopsy surgery.

I was able to convince him to do another biopsy surgery. After the first one (performed before I started treatment), I was not a fan of doing it again; this could be called a hollow victory.

Before the surgery, my surgeon (this is a different surgeon than the one that did the first biopsy) said he was sure nothing was wrong. After the surgery, my surgeon again said he was certain nothing was wrong. I just had to wait for the lab tests to come back.

"Yes, you are cured of cancer."

The lab test came back from the biopsy and showed no cancer. I emailed the surgeon, asking if this meant I was cured of cancer. One of his staff responded, stating that the surgeon said, "Yes, you are cured of cancer."

"Why am I not feeling better, Doctor?" The 2nd ENT responded, "I Don't Know." The doctor did not seem concerned.

A few months after my second biopsy surgery, I was in my radiologist's exam room to be scoped.

This was the last time I saw that radiologist; she was in a hurry (they were having a staff meeting with free sandwiches). She started our exam by saying I was doing so well that I no longer needed to be scoped every month; I should now get scoped every other month. I felt like hell.

The scope was not working. My radiologist got a different scope, where only she could see what was happening (no video monitor). She is looking down my throat with one of her legs out the door (the free sandwiches were calling, just kidding).

She stops and says, "You are not symmetrical!" I was amazed at the amount of concern in her voice. I have been called several things, some valid, but I have never been accused of being "not symmetrical." I was not sure what she meant. She kept repeating the exact words, "not symmetrical." She changes lenses on the scope and goes up and down the throat.

"You need to see your surgeon; I'll call him today." I was never told what she meant. I had a good idea of what she meant.

Going into the **third** surgery with the 2nd ENT, the surgeon told my niece and me he was sure there was no cancer. After the surgery, the surgeon reiterated that there was no cancer. The biopsies were sent to the lab for analysis.

You are Not cured; it is back (actually, it never left)

Doctors sometimes talk in a manner that is not intelligible. The result of tests is an excellent example. The biopsy came back positive. In

English, the word positive is a good thing. In this situation, it is a terrible thing.

When I received the test result, and the test was positive, I had to make sure I told myself, "Positive is a bad thing."

Not a surprise to me; I knew I was not feeling well. I do not understand why doctors do not understand if the patient is not feeling well; the patient is sick.

I hate it when I am right, especially when it means dying.

They did another PET scan.

I'm sitting in my 2nd ENT exam room. I had been given the biopsy report by email. I knew the bad part, I thought.

Biopsies were taken in an area smaller than the area of a quarter. The cancer was everywhere. There was so much of it; it was nearly impossible for the surgeon to miss it this time.

Asking the top Face Neck surgeon in Huston, TX (see Chapter 13) about the second biopsy where they found nothing wrong, he said they probably just missed cancer [too small of an area taken].

The 2nd ENT said I would have to do a massive neck reconstruction. The result means I may be unable to eat, drink, swallow, or speak. I might be able to sit up all day and watch television.

"Breathe."

While the doctor gave me this news, my apple watch shook my wrist. I looked down at my watch, and it said, "Breathe." I almost cracked a smile while getting the worst news of my life.

Probably the only reason I did not crack a smile as I was afraid I would have been sent to the nut house if I did smile. I liked my watch after that; my watch had the same obtuse sense of humor I had.

Humor is wherever you wish to find it. Things are not funny only if you choose them to be not funny. A colossal belly laugh can make horrible news tolerable.

The doctor ended our meeting by saying surgery is the best option, but there is a new drug that will probably not work.

My Oncologist, my healthcare provider, told me they usually don't do surgery on a patient if it will not save their life. They would do surgery on me to give me some comfort from the pain. The previous biopsy surgeries were excruciating; the comfort surgery would be much more invasive (it will hurt a lot).

When I got home, I immediately called my surgeon and requested a referral to talk to a doctor about the new drug.

I saw an oncologist about the drug. He said he would have to get special permission from the FDA (Food and Drug Administration) under the "Drug as of Last Resort" act. The FDA would only approve it if I had no other course of action.

The drug was not approved for my type of cancer. Since everything else had failed, I might be able to get the drug.

To see if there were other options, the next day, I headed to the top cancer clinic in the world based in Houston, Texas.

What I learned from Chapter 12:

As a patient, you are the customer. The customer is always right.

If you don't feel well, tell your doctor. Keep telling your doctor until your doctor understands you are ill.

Keep insisting until you get what you want. Never give up.

13: Houston, Texas

I fly to Houston, Texas, the location of the top cancer institute in the world. My last hope. This clinic is about eighteen stories tall, and all floors were filled with cancer patients.

I hand them a check for thirty-thousand dollars. I then meet with the head surgeon and his staff. The head surgeon orders them to run all of the tests.

After all their tests, I again meet with the head surgeon and his primary staff (all doctors).

He shows me their scans.

Seeing the scans, I say, "No robotic surgery." The doctor responded, "That's correct."

My primary care 2nd ENT told me that robotic surgery was unacceptable since my mouth was too small. And that robotic surgery was not as good as regular surgery. Regular surgery would require massive rebuilding of my throat, possibly leaving me unable to swallow, talk, eat, etc.

Houston, TX clinic told me my mouth was Not too small, and robotic surgery was far Superior to regular surgery because it did far less damage if you have experience with robotic surgery. They said the only limiting factor would be if cancer spread too much.

Cancer had spread too much for robotic surgery, so no robotic surgery.

He shows me more of the scan.

I say, "No surgery."

The doctor says, 'We don't recommend it." The meeting was over. The only possibility of surgery was if the cancer mass was reduced.

This is how I was told to "go home and die." We said (my sister was with me in Houston), "thank you," and left. I could give up now, go home, and die. That is not going to happen.

At our initial meeting, I had told the Houston, TX surgeon that dancing was my life; it was my only form of exercise and my single social outlet. That played into the diagnosis of not doing any surgery on me.

I meet with an oncologist in Houston's clinic. She suggested I become part of a study where they use the same drug my healthcare provider, my oncologist, was asking permission to use on me from the FDA. The Houston clinic would only give me two doses of this drug, then perform surgery.

If you don't give up, you will never lose.

My healthcare provider's oncologist called while I was in Texas. The FDA had approved me to try the Drug. My healthcare provider had agreed to nine doses of this drug. My previous discussion with this doctor was if it does not work, you will probably die. Cancer would likely spread too much by the end of the treatment.

I flew into LAX (Los Angeles airport) the next day and took an Uber home. I cleaned up, took a nap, and went dancing. While in Texas, finding a place to ballroom dance was not easy. I found one; I went once. I needed to dance.

<u>I start the drug in a week.</u>

The speed is a nice change. The FDA approved me for this drug in less than two weeks. Houston, TX, told me what I had in less than a week and mentioned several things my healthcare provider did wrong (no big surprise on the wrong stuff).

What I learned from Chapter 13:

Just because a doctor or institution is the best does not mean they have the right solution for you. Go for the best solution for you, but trust but verify.

14: Revelation

During my chemo & radiation treatment, I still went dancing a few times. Pre-illness I would dance two to three times a week. During chemo & radiation treatment, I danced three times over two months. One of the times was just for 30 minutes.

After the initial treatment (chemo & radiation) was completed, I eventually danced twice a week, even though I was not feeling good.

My oncologist was talking to me about this drug that might help some. He said, "If it does not work, at least you've lived a good life." When he said that to me, I felt like punching him in the face.

Oncologist works with ill people; some of them are about to die. He was not trying to be mean. He stated the facts as he saw them. He did not know me; he did not know what type of life I had lived.

I was upset because he was wrong; I had not lived a good life. I am not an evil person or a mean person. I put a very high standard of morals in my life. Thinking through why I was so mad at my oncologist, I realized I was missing something big. If the doctors were right, I had no time to correct my life positively.

There was something wrong with my life besides my dying.

The Doctor is an Oncologist who works with cancer. He is in the department that does Chemo Therapy. Most people think chemotherapy is all cancer patients getting an IV to kill cancer. Chemo is indeed delivered via IV. Chemo is a specific set of drugs; that defines how they work on the body. Not all cancer drugs are chemo drugs.

Technically it is called infusion when giving a drug via IV. I have heard the drug I was getting was called chemo, which is incorrect. It was immunology therapy. It is changing your immune system to fight cancer instead of a drug trying to kill cancer directly.

I was approved for nine doses. One dose every three weeks with a blood test up to three days before each infusion.

My throat was feeling bad. I was scheduled for a PET scan after the fourth treatment. A PET scan is where you are injected with radioactive sugar. My type of cancer is like sugar. The radioactive sugar is attracted to cancer. The scanner locates where the radioactive sugar is situated. This is very accurate in finding this type of cancer. The only problem is injecting a person with more radiation that has had 70 grays of radiation therapy is unhealthy.

Before the PET scan results, I would wake up in the middle of the night and think about what I would accept.

> I will accept if the cancer is reduced (not likely). This would mean I could have surgery to remove the rest of cancer and maybe have a decent quality of life.

> I would accept that cancer had not grown. Not a great situation; at least I would have more time to live. Maybe if I stayed on the drug, it would not grow anymore. Acceptable situation.

> If cancer had grown, I would be dying soon. Nothing could be done for me. I

could try to find another new drug. I had already started the research.

I had a PET scan right after the fourth dose of the drug. I waited and danced for a long ten days to get the results. I was having pain in my neck. When I told my Oncologist about the pain, he told me to be prepared for the worse.

What I learned from Chapter 14:

Sometimes you have to make a decision that is not based on the percentages but on what type of life you want. I had thought luck was not part of your treatment determination.

You might have to hope for luck, religion, or intelligent decision. Or possibly a little of all of the above.

15: The End?

I get checked in to meet with my doctor (oncologist). I told the nurse that I was not expecting a good result. My neck had been feeling horrible. The doctor picks me up at the nurse's station. Unusual, usually, a nurse takes me to an exam room and leaves me there waiting for a doctor to show up.

I walk with my doctor in what seems to be a very long hallway. I had never been this far down this hallway. We get to a room; it does not seem to be a regular exam room (more of a storage room). The doctor logs onto the computer. The doctor shows me previous and current PET scans and quickly flips back and forth.

Sometimes being wrong can be right.

I was half in shock, having trouble processing the pictures. Was this the end of my life? What was my doctor showing me?

My doctor then gave me the cancer cell count (I did not know they could count the number of cancer cells). The count was drastically lower now than in the previous scan. I asked, "My cancer has been reduced by 75%?" My doctor did not answer the question. We talked for a minute or two. He walked me back to the nurse's station so she could check me out.

I later realized my math was wrong; it was closer to a reduction of 70%.

I started to tell the nurse what had happened. I ask for a tissue. She hands me a small box. I break down, standing in the nurse's station.

The nurse left, saying to take as long as I needed. I stood there, crying for about 10 seconds.

I am a guy; we do not cry, we do not cry in public, and we do not cry on good news. I went home and called everyone I knew. The drug that had almost no chance of working worked far better than 'everyone' thought possible.

About a week later, I was in again for another infusion. My doctor stops by and asks, "I guess you are ready to go to surgery [to remove the rest of cancer]?" The plan at the Huston, TX clinic was two doses, then surgery. At my healthcare provider, it was nine doses, then surgery. The drug was supposed to reduce the tumor only if it worked at all slightly.

My response to my doctor's query has changed many people's lives, including mine. I said, "Why stop getting the drug if it works?" My doctor stares at me for a few seconds, turns, and walks away without saying a word.

Even minor surgery could cause drastic changes. The changes were a long list of things that were unacceptable to me. No surgery meant that I would have an everyday life.

I go to San Diego to see a surgeon who used to work at the Huston, TX clinic. He looks me over with a scope and says he saw no evidence of cancer. He believes the PET scan was taken too soon after my previous infusion, so the last Drug did not have time to work. He said I was probably cancer-free. I like the good news. I was positive he was correct.

I danced for four days a week. I felt great.

I was positive he was correct, but I still had my fingers crossed for luck.

After the ninth treatment, I had another PET scan. I was sure it would show no cancer. I was correct.

I love it when I am right when it means I will live.

I showed no cancer. But the party is not over. Scans are not perfect, nor can they show small amounts of cancer just hanging out, ready to grow again rapidly.

My doctor told me I might be on the drug for a year or two, three, or maybe forever. I scoffed at the idea that I would be on the drug forever. I need to pay attention to the deals I make with myself. Staying on the drug was one of the acceptable options.

I was the first patient on this drug for throat cancer for this healthcare provider. I have been on the drug for almost two years. I get scoped every few months. I insisted on being scoped every two months. I tolerate endoscopes as just part of my life.

I have had complex discussions with my doctors about when I should have my following PET scan. I need to know if the cancer returns, but the PET scans' radiation could cause cancer.

I have had many life decisions in the past six years. I am sure my being alive is more luck than smarts or bravery.

I know with certainty that more people are alive because I took a chance on the drug when I asked: "Why Stop?"

The FDA has approved the drug for use on my type of cancer after my success with the drug.

I was told by a nurse that "a lot" of her patients with my same type of cancer are now getting my drug. The drug has been approved as the first line of treatment; no radiation treatment is required.

Each day I get up and say no to a PET scan today because I feel great; it is a decision I will live with until tomorrow.

What I learned from Chapter 15:

At some point, everything will go right. Belief in a good result will help you get through the process.

16: Now What?

The old comedic actor W. C. Fields was known to have said, "I'd never join a club that would have me as a member."

I wondered what type of woman would want a man fighting cancer. Surprisingly, I found out that there was more than one.

I was now not fighting against cancer daily; after the fourth dose, when I got the news that the drug was working. My mind turns to women, not that they were ever completely out of my mind.

I had a girlfriend that knew about my cancer. She seemed fine with the idea. She said her sister had cancer ten years ago and is healthy now.

The attitude changed when I told her about my conversation with the doctor when he mentioned that I could be on the drug forever. I am unsure if that was the reason, the straw that broke the camel's back, or something utterly foreign to the cancer problem. She sent me a note that she did not want to marry me. I have not seen her since then (over two years ago).

An Infusion Nurse (the nurse in the chemo department) told me that it is not uncommon to hear about breakups caused by cancer.

I have lectured over half the world on computer systems. My intelligence is above average, but I do not think I will completely understand women. I think women prefer it that way.

Any pain in my neck region causes me to stop and sweat a little.

The doctor told me that a nurse sometimes said drugs stop working. Something that rings in my ear from time to time. I could sit around worrying about what would happen if this drug stopped working. I think it is better to get my life plan in order. I am more likely to die from walking in front of a bus than from cancer.

I was utterly dedicated to recovering from cancer and not dying for the past six years.

Dance, dance, dance and program, program, program, and write a few more books. And hopefully, someday, have someone with which to enjoy life.

I am working on setting my life's goals. Goals are done when you are 15, 20, or 25 years old. Being uncertain about what to do after surviving cancer is not unusual. Your full time is devoted to cancer; if you are cured, then what?

Currently, one absolute every three weeks, a blood draw, then an infusion. I wouldn't say I like getting stuck two times every three weeks, but I am not giving up.

What I learned from Chapter 16:

You are a person, not a disease. Do not let anyone label you the "cancer person." You are who you are, whether you have the flu or cancer.

The world runs the same way before you had cancer and will run the same way after you are cured.

17: It Is Your Fault

My oncologist came into the infusion room where I was receiving the Drug. In an accusatory tone (think Perry Mason) and says, "people are dying on your drug!"

I considered this Drug as my Drug. I felt all of my pain and suffering was worth it since it had the possibility of helping many people.

I felt very guilty that people were dying on my drug. I did not create the drug or administer the drug. But I thought this drug could be used as the only treatment needed to cure my type of cancer.

Previously, doctors thought the Drug would only be helpful as a treatment before surgery. This Drug would allow advanced cancer patients to have surgery that otherwise had no options.

I rarely saw my Oncologist; everything was going smoothly, and there was no reason to see him. The last two times I saw him, he was delighted and said, "You are making me look good."

After their success with me, he started to use the drug on other patients. The next person dies. My Oncologist said it was because his cancer was so advanced.

My cancer was very advanced when they started to use it on me. My cancer was at Stage 5, the worse that it could get.

From my Oncologist's anger, it was apparent they were using it on several more patients.

It was later found that the first Chemo drug I had one dose of was the reason the Drug worked.

The FDA has approved the Drug to be the only treatment for my type of cancer when given the Chemo drug.

One would think that everything would be great between my Oncologist and me. It was not.

He started asking me to stop using the drug. The first reason he gave was that it cost too much.

I said no. The next time I was in for infusion, I heard my oncologist talking to my infusion nurse in the hallway.

I get almost every infusion from a different nurse.

Today's infusion nurse came into my infusion room and discussed the drug's expense. She gave a different dollar amount than my Oncologist.

Usually, doctors and nurses do not know and are not concerned about drug costs.

I started traveling around talking to other Oncologists about whether to stop using the drug. Every time I meet a new doctor (not just Oncologists, but all doctors), the scene would go like this, the doctor would come into the room and say, "Hello Geoffrey, my name is [fill in the blank]" They would sit down turn to look at me and say, "Wow."

I did not notice the Wow for the first couple of doctors until the third time it happened.

Since this Drug was new, no doctor would say when was a good time to stop using it.

I called the Drug manufacturer; they would not say when it would be a good time to stop. The Drug company started to call me every month to see if I was doing Okay.

The Drug company sent me a hundred-page report in fine print on the studies they had done on the report. The trials only lasted for two years.

I started reading all medical articles I could find on the Drug.

The EU (European Union) tried a different dosage where the patient got an infusion every six weeks instead of every three weeks. I was getting it every three weeks.

I asked to get the higher dosage every six weeks.

My Oncologist said it cost too much more. He said the three-week dosage cost $50,000, and the six-week dosage was $75,000.

I said, "Management is a bunch of F***ing idiots!"

To cover six weeks, two doses of the three-week would cost $100,000, while the six-week would cost $75,000.

My Oncologist said he would tell management what I said.

They switched me to the six-week dose with no additional side effects. They saved more on blood tests, nurse time, and doctor time (about 5 minutes a month).

No "thank you" from my healthcare provider for saving them money.

A few months later, looking at the Drug's website created by the Drug company said the Drug costs about $1,100. That is a big difference from what I was told.

What I learned from Chapter 17:

What your doctor may tell you may not be correct.
Trust but verify.

18: Eight rules to a Successful Life

I was describing the new toilet I had put in my place to a friend. He says wow, you are really happy. I was smiling about a toilet. It had been years since I could say that I looked happy. A toilet had nothing to do with my happiness.

The toilet was nothing special, your basic white dual flush toilet. I had never installed one before, so I enjoyed the accomplishment. I enjoy accomplishing something I have not done before. I also enjoyed taking a sludge hammer to the old ugly yellow toilet. That was fun.

Most people who do their renovation enjoy the most the destruction part. It is hard to make a mistake when you are destroying something. Unless it is a wall you are demolishing and you went too far.

I am happy.

Writing this book, I had not planned on this chapter. Getting close to the end of the book, I noticed several things that kept determining my life—whether I am alive or not, whether I am happy or not. Below I found my life's rules over the past six years. These rules can help you.

1. If you don't know where you are going (your goal), you can't get there.

The above is one of my favorite sayings about business life that I should have applied to my life. I never set a grand goal for my life.

Getting rich is not a goal (it is a side effect). Not having a destination is like getting the family into the car and starting driving. The kids start asking, "Are we there yet?" You cannot answer because you do not know where you are going.

Your destination is more important than yoga, a new car, creating a list, or the weather. Find your destination; everything else is strictly secondary to establishing your goal.

Over the past six years, my destination has been not to die. I now need a new destination with plenty of laughter and smiles. It is like starting over in college. Everything is possible; you have to decide what you want.

Some may find it challenging to decide on such importance. If so, ask your spouse or best friend what they think should be your goal. If they are no help, write down every possible goal and put it in the hat. Pick one out of the hat and go for it. Select another goal if you find out later it is not what you want. Please do not pick a new goal every week. Give your goal a chance to get embedded into your life before throwing that goal out.

To help you determine if something you want as a goal, think of yourself in the future, in your rocking chair, talking to your grandchildren (it does not matter if you don't want children, this is a mental exercise). You are telling your grandchildren about your fabulous life. What do you tell them you accomplished? That is your goal.

2. If you don't give up, you will never lose.

It seems obvious but giving up means defeat; for me, it meant death.

In obtaining your goals, you need to try again and then try again. There is no limit on how many times you try except for an arbitrary number set by you. Throughout life, you may change your goal or destination. Getting married and having kids will adjust your goal. A new job in a new town can have the same effect.

If you are starting but never complete working on your goal, you are probably trying to achieve too much too fast.

Suppose you are getting sick of your goal. Most people find it difficult to change old habits and try something new.

A solution I found to help me get going on a goal I keep putting off is to work on your goal for at least two minutes every day. This method (taken from Kaizen) is what the Japanese use for working on a hard or tedious task. Of course, you can work longer than two minutes. Every day you do have two minutes to work on your goal. Everyone has two minutes extra in their life. You have no excuses, so get to work.

If your goal is not dying, spend more than two minutes daily.

By taking one little step at a time, you will move on to the path to achieving your goal. You will get used to working on your goal and find yourself quickly increasing the time you spend on it.

3. Attitude determines whether you enjoy life or do not enjoy life.

When I started my professional life, I used to fly all over the United States. On a lecture tour, I flew all over Central America and South America. Bad turbulence I took as just bumps in the road. My attitude changed one day on a flight from Southern California to Northern California. The turbulence was terrible, but I have been through worse. I had recently read several articles on airline crashes.

I had a death grip on the armrests; I was sure the plane would crash, and there would be nothing. I would no longer exist. "Fade to black," as they say in Hollywood.

I did continue flying after that bad flight; I flew less and did not enjoy it. I should have learned a life lesson. Flying was something I enjoyed; now I hate it, and the only difference is my change of attitude toward flying. It was not less safe to fly; planes were not falling out of the sky, planes were not less comfortable, and the flight attendants were just as nice (most of them). Only my attitude had changed. Flying went from luxury, fun, and enjoyable to something dreaded.

I have gotten better about flying but do not get the joy it used to bring me.

Some people enjoy an evening rain; some dread it. Some people enjoy a bird singing, while others wish it to shut up so they can get some rest.

You are the one that determines if you are enjoying your life.

Attitude is everything for things that you interface with often. For situations, you do not like to find a reason to like them.

The goofy secretary counts the number of times they smack their gum. Such habits can be a good indicator of mood. Be a detective and try to figure out what each count means.

The crazy business partner that drives you nuts overdoing everything in a very formal slow manner. Find the humor in the situation. Humor can cure most of these situations, so laugh.

Every day you determine if it is a good day.

4. **Anger can be a good thing.**

We all have been told that anger is a bad thing. That anger can make you do bad things.

Anger is not necessarily destructive but a reaction to a bad situation. It is terrible if the anger is so intense it immobilizes you or causes you to do bad things. Please make sure you note the difference between good anger and destructive anger.

If you become angry for little or no cause, that is bad anger.

Anger is a strong emotion; if anger is directed in the correct direction, it can be beneficial. Instead of freezing in place, it gives you the ability to move.

Instead of whining that I was going to die, I used the anger about the horrible medical help to direct my emotions elsewhere. The rage enabled me to make the correct decisions about my care. I did not accept the situation as presented to me.

Anger is our strongest emotion. It can be used to your benefit if you control it. Or it could destroy your life. Make sure you understand the difference between good and bad emotions. When anger is used correctly, it can help you reach your goal.

We all have times when we are angry in life. As long as you control it, you will be fine.

5. **Humor can be a great weapon.**"Breathe."

Humor is wherever you wish to find it. Things are not funny if you choose them to be not funny. A huge belly laugh can make horrible news tolerable.

I had difficulty not smiling when getting the worse news of my life when my watch told me to breathe. Maybe I should have laughed; big deal if the doctor thought I was a nut. The right attitude meant I made the right decision (try the drug and not the surgery).

Everything in life should be able to bring a smile to your face. We are trained not to smile at certain times. It may sometimes be inappropriate, but it will make you feel good.

Try smiling or laughing aloud the next time you are at a funeral. Probably a good idea to bring along a humorous story about the deceased. The story will help you stay out of the asylum.

If you are fired from your perfect job, try laughing aloud to your supervisor. If it does not save your job for you or get you more parting money, it will put you in a mood to go out and immediately get a better job (the situation was not all that perfect if you got fired from it).

In such situations, remember never to burn your

bridges. Do not tell your boss what you think about him. What if the firing was a mistake, but now you cannot return? How you leave your old job will make the difference between getting and not getting a new job.

Not just your supervisor/boss; treat every person in the world like you may need their help sometime in the future. You will have more friends, and maybe one of them will be a doctor.

6. If you are not feeling well, but the doctor is not helping you feel better. Find a new doctor.

This rule goes for more than doctors; it goes for any professional. If they are not doing their job, get someone else. Life is short. Make the best of life by not dealing with the incompetents and stupid people of the world.

If your mechanic does not fix the problem, find a new mechanic. If the fast-food restaurant keeps getting your order wrong, go to a different one (millions of them).

Talk to your doctor about your concerns when your family or friends say how you are being treated poorly. If no change comes from the conversation, find a new doctor. There are about as many doctors as there are fast-food joints.

Every time you see your doctor, even for minor problems, your life is in their hands. Maintain a watch over your doctor, and you will be happier and healthier.

Remember, "Trust but Verify."

7. **I love it when I am right when it means I will live.**

Remember to enjoy your victories because life is not all victories. If your wife creates a good meal, you are awarded the Medal of Honor, caught that green light, or elected President. Enjoy it. It keeps you grounded in what is essential to your life.

Celebrate the victory for several days until a new win comes. There are a lot of green lights to catch.

Looking for things to celebrate can change your life for the better. Looking for the good is far better for your attitude than remembering the bad.

Come home happy from work because you caught four green lights. Celebrating a green light is better than coming home angry because some jerk cut you off.

Take it even further and think of good things that could happen today. Celebrate those thoughts. It will put you in a great attitude and make your day more productive.

Attitude is especially crucial if you are fighting for your life. Talking to your medical professionals with a good view will always improve your results.

I joke with the nurse or technician about poking

me with a needle. I also make a point of telling them how painful the needle pokes are to me. You will get the least amount of pain that is possible if you nicely talk to them.

8. **Just because someone is excellent at their job does not mean they are always right.**

No matter how good someone is at their job, they can make mistakes. Always keep your eyes wide open. "Trust but verify."

My top-of-the-line Realtor was wrong about when to sell my condo. Her other actions have all been excellent. "Trust but verify."

Use the top talent you can find, but "Trust but verify."

Price is not a good indicator of whether a person is excellent at their job. Remember to verify the reputation before paying top dollar. You will usually save money long-term and be less frustrated with the outcome.

Doctors come in all flavors, some good, some bad, some concerned, and some could care less.

I do not think (at least I hope) my experience is not typical of all doctors. Some of the problems came from the healthcare providers trying to convert the doctors into conveyor belts that push patients through as fast as possible, not having time to get to know the patient or their problem.

One doctor at my healthcare provider told me he

had over a thousand patients. It took at least two months to see him, which is typical for all doctors at my provider. Healthcare management seems to know how to cut costs but has no idea how patients need to be treated.

19: Stress

Stress may have contributed to the development of cancer. The reduction of stress for the patient might greatly help with the cure of cancer.

The patient and those close to the patient (family or friends) must reduce their stress level.

Stress is a natural physical and emotional response to life experiences. When you feel threatened, your body's defenses kick into high gear in a rapid, automatic "fight-or-flight" response. The fight-or-flight response is your body's way of protecting you. It happens when you sense danger and prepares your body to either fight or take off running. This response is triggered by the release of hormones such as adrenaline, which gives you energy and strength.

Various factors, such as serious illness, work, relationships, and financial problems, can cause stress. It is a normal part of life, but if you experience anxiety regularly can take a toll on your physical and emotional health. Chronic stress can lead to various health problems, such as high blood pressure, heart disease, and depression. Finding healthy ways to manage stress is essential, such as exercising, relaxation techniques, and getting enough sleep.

Patients, family members, and friends of the patient need to realize the importance of reducing stress. Stressed family members and friends will cause increased pressure on the patient.

So everyone should be practicing at least one of the stress reduction techniques mentioned in this chapter.

Things that Cause Stress

Many things can cause stress, and what causes pressure can vary significantly from person to person. Some common causes of stress include:

1. Work: Job pressure, long hours, and difficult coworkers or bosses can all be sources of stress.
2. Relationships: Difficult or strained relationships with family, friends, or a significant other can cause stress.
3. Finances: Money problems, such as struggling to pay bills or being in debt, can be a significant source of stress.
4. Health: Chronic health problems or the fear of developing a health condition can cause stress.
5. Life changes: Major life changes, such as moving, getting married, or starting a family, can be stressful.

6. Personal problems: Stress can be caused by emotional problems, such as low self-esteem or lack of fulfillment.
7. The environment: Noise, pollution, and a cluttered environment can contribute to stress.
8. Trauma: Past trauma, such as abuse or losing a loved one, can cause stress.
9. Burnout: When you feel overwhelmed and unable to meet the demands of your life, it can lead to burnout and stress.

Good and Bad Stress

Some evidence suggests that chronic stress may play a role in developing certain types of cancer.

Chronic stress has been linked to an increased risk of specific health problems, such as high blood pressure, heart disease, and weakened immune function, which may increase cancer risk.

However, it's important to note that stress is just one of many factors that can influence cancer risk. Other factors, such as genetics, diet, and exposure to certain substances, also play a role.

It's also worth noting that stress is a normal part of life, and not all stress is harmful. Short-term stress, such as the kind you might experience during a deadline at work or a difficult conversation, is a normal and healthy part of life. Chronic stress or stress that persists over a long time can be more harmful.

Speaking with a healthcare professional is a good idea if you're experiencing chronic stress and are concerned about your health. They can help you identify the causes of your stress and recommend strategies for managing it.

Ways to Reduce Stress

There are many ways to reduce stress, and what works for one person may not work for another. Here are a few ideas that might help:

1. Exercise regularly. Physical activity can help reduce stress by releasing endorphins, chemicals that improve mood and reduce feelings of stress and anxiety.

Many exercises can help reduce stress; the best one for you depends on your preferences and fitness level. Some good options include:

A. Aerobic exercise: Activities such as running, cycling, and swimming can help reduce stress by releasing endorphins and providing a sense of accomplishment.

B. Yoga: This mind-body practice involves physical poses, deep breathing, and meditation and has been shown to reduce stress and improve mood.

C. Tai chi: This low-impact martial art involves gentle, flowing movements and deep breathing and is a good option for people of all ages and fitness levels.

D. Strength training: Lifting weights or doing other types of strength training can help reduce stress by providing a sense of accomplishment and boosting self-confidence.

E. Outdoor activities: Getting out into nature can help reduce stress and improve mood. Options might include hiking, gardening, or even just going for a walk.

Ultimately, the most important thing is to find an exercise you enjoy and can make a part of your routine. This will make it more likely that you'll stick with it and get the stress-reducing benefits.

2. Get enough sleep. Lack of sleep can increase stress, so you must ensure you're getting enough rest.

There are several things you can try to increase the amount of time you sleep:

A. Stick to a consistent sleep schedule: Try to go to bed and wake up at the same time every day, even on weekends. A schedule can help regulate your body's natural sleep-wake cycle.

B. Create a sleep-friendly environment: Keep your bedroom dark, calm, and quiet, and invest in a comfortable mattress and pillows.

C. Wind down before bed: Avoid screens (phone, computer, TV) and other stimulating activities for at least an hour before bedtime.

Instead, try reading, listening to soothing music, or taking a warm bath.

D. Avoid caffeine and alcohol close to bedtime: Both substances can disrupt sleep. It's best to avoid them, especially in the hours leading up to bedtime.

E. Exercise regularly: Regular physical activity can help you fall asleep more quickly and sleep more soundly. Just be sure to finish your workout a few hours before bed, as exercise can also be a stimulant.

F. Eat a healthy diet: A well-balanced diet can help promote good sleep, so try to eat various nutritious foods and avoid going to bed hungry or overly full.

G. Avoid napping: Napping during the day can interfere with your ability to fall asleep at night. If you're feeling tired, try to push through and get some rest that night.

H. Get some sunlight: Exposure to sunlight during the day can help regulate your body's natural sleep-wake cycle and improve your sleep quality.

I. Consider relaxation techniques: Techniques such as deep breathing, meditation, or progressive muscle relaxation can help calm the mind and body and prepare you for sleep.

J. Talk to your doctor: If you're having trouble sleeping, speaking with a healthcare professional is a good idea. They can help you identify any underlying issues and recommend treatment options if necessary.

K. Eat a healthy diet. A well-balanced diet can help you feel better physically, which can, in turn, help reduce stress.

L. Take breaks and engage in activities you enjoy. Make time for leisure activities and hobbies that you find enjoyable and relaxing.

M. Seek social support. Talk to friends and family, or consider joining a support group. Sharing your feelings and concerns with others can help reduce stress.

N. Set realistic goals. Trying to do too much can lead to stress, so it's important to set achievable goals.

O. Learn to manage your time effectively. Planning and prioritizing your tasks can help reduce the feeling of being overwhelmed.

P. Try stress-reducing activities such as massage or aromatherapy. These can help relax the body and mind.

Q. Seek professional help if your stress is severe or persistent. A mental health professional can help you identify the causes of your stress and develop strategies for managing it.

R. Eat a healthy diet. A well-balanced diet can help you feel better physically, which can, in turn, help reduce stress.

3. Stress-reducing diets may help. There is no one "stress-reducing" diet that works for everyone, but there are some general dietary principles that can help reduce stress and improve overall well-being:

A. Eat a varied diet with plenty of fruits, vegetables, whole grains, and lean proteins. These foods provide the nutrients your body needs to function optimally.

B. Limit your intake of sugary and processed foods, which can cause fluctuations in blood sugar levels and contribute to feelings of stress and anxiety.

C. Stay hydrated by drinking plenty of water throughout the day.

Dehydration can contribute to feelings of fatigue and stress.

D. Consider incorporating stress-reducing foods into your diet. Some options include:

* Foods high in antioxidants, such as berries and leafy greens, which can help

protect against the adverse effects of stress on the body

* Foods rich in omega-3 fatty acids, such as fatty fish and flaxseeds, which have been shown to have anti-inflammatory effects and may help reduce stress and improve mood

* Foods containing vitamin C, such as citrus fruits and bell peppers, which may help reduce the effects of stress on the body

E. Don't skip meals, especially breakfast. Skipping meals can lead to low blood sugar levels, which can cause feelings of stress and anxiety.

F. Consider using herbs and spices to add flavor to your meals. Some herbs and spices, such as basil, chamomile, and ginger, have been shown to have stress-reducing properties.

It's important to remember that everyone is different, and what works for one person may not work for another. Experimenting with different approaches to see what works best for you is a good idea.

4. Take breaks and engage in activities you enjoy. Make time for leisure activities and hobbies that you find enjoyable and relaxing.

Many leisure activities can help reduce stress and improve overall well-being. Some good options include:

A. Exercise: Physical activity can help reduce stress by releasing endorphins, chemicals that improve mood and reduce feelings of stress and anxiety.

B. Hobbies: Engaging in hobbies and activities you enjoy, such as painting, cooking, or gardening, can provide a sense of accomplishment and help take your mind off of stressors.

C. Reading: Curling up with a good book can be relaxing and enjoyable to unwind.

D. Outdoor activities: Getting out into nature can help reduce stress and improve mood. Options might include hiking, biking, or just going for a walk.

E. Social activities: Spending time with friends and loved ones can help reduce stress and improve overall well-being.

F. Relaxation techniques: Techniques such as deep breathing, meditation, and yoga can help calm the mind and body.

G. Spa treatments: Massages and facials can help relax the mind and body and provide a sense of pampering and indulgence.

It's essential to find leisure activities you enjoy and can be part of your routine. This will make it more likely that you'll stick with them and get the stress-reducing benefits.

5. Seek social support. Talk to friends and family, or consider joining a support group. Sharing your feelings and concerns with others can help reduce stress.

Social support can be a powerful tool for reducing stress and improving overall well-being. Here are a few ways to get social support:

A. Talk to friends and family: Sharing your feelings and concerns with trusted loved ones can significantly reduce stress and make you feel more connected.

B. Join a support group: Support groups can provide a sense of community and a safe space to share your feelings and experiences with others who are going through similar challenges.

C. Seek out a mentor or coach: Having someone to turn to for guidance and support can be beneficial in reducing stress and achieving your goals.

D. Volunteer: Helping others can be a great way to feel more connected and purposeful, which can, in turn, help reduce stress.

E. Connect with others online: There are many online communities and forums where you can connect and share your experiences.

Just be sure to use these resources responsibly and protect your personal information.

It's important to remember that social support is not a one-size-fits-all solution, and what works for one person may not work for another. Experiment with different ways of getting social support to find what works best for you.

6. Set realistic goals. Trying to do too much can lead to stress, so it's essential to set achievable goals.

Setting realistic goals can help reduce stress and improve your chances of success. Here are a few tips for setting realistic goals:

A. Start by setting small, achievable goals. The goals can help build momentum and confidence as you work towards larger objectives.

B. Clearly define your goals. Make sure your goals are specific, measurable, attainable, relevant, and time-bound (SMART goals). Plans will help you stay focused and make progress.

C. Be realistic about what you can accomplish. Don't try to take on too much at once. Instead, focus on a few key goals that you can realistically achieve.

D. Break your goals down into smaller, more manageable tasks. This can help make the goal feel more achievable and help you make progress.

E. Make a plan and stick to it. Identify the steps you need to take to achieve your goals, and allocate time and resources accordingly.

F. Keep track of your progress. This can help you stay motivated and see how far you've come.

G. Be flexible. Life can be unpredictable, so be prepared to adjust your plans as needed.

8. Celebrate your successes. Take time to recognize and appreciate your accomplishments, big and small.

Remember, setting and achieving goals is a process that takes time and effort. Be patient with yourself, and don't be afraid to ask for help when you need it.

7. Learn to manage your time effectively. Planning and prioritizing your tasks can help reduce the feeling of being overwhelmed.

Effective time management can help reduce stress and improve your well-being. Here are a few tips for managing your time:

A. Set priorities: Identify the most critical tasks on your to-do list and focus on them first.

B. Create a schedule: Break your day into blocks of time and allocate specific tasks to each block. This can help you stay focused and on track.

C. Limit distractions: Turn off notifications on your phone and computer, and create a quiet, distraction-free workspace.

D. Take breaks: It's important to rest and recharge.

Schedule regular breaks into your day to help you stay energized and focused.

E. Delegate tasks: Don't hesitate to ask for help or delegate tasks to others. This can help you manage your time more effectively and reduce overwhelming feelings.

F. Avoid multitasking: Focusing on one task at a time can help you work more efficiently and reduce stress.

G. Practice saying "no": It's okay to say no to requests or commitments that don't align with your priorities or that would stretch you too thin.

H. Seek out time-saving tools and resources: Many tools and resources are available to help you manage your time more effectively.

Experiment with different options to find what works best for you. Effectively managing your time takes practice, but with a little effort, you can develop strategies and habits that help you feel more in control and reduce stress.

8. Try stress-reducing activities such as massage or aromatherapy. These can help relax the body and mind.

There are many stress-reducing activities that you can try, and the best one for you will depend on your personal preferences and lifestyle. Here are a few ideas:

A. Exercise: Physical activity can help reduce stress by releasing endorphins, chemicals that improve mood and reduce feelings of stress and anxiety.

B. Practice relaxation techniques: Techniques such as deep breathing, meditation, and yoga can help calm the mind and body.

C. Spend time in nature: Getting out into nature can help reduce stress and improve mood. Options might include hiking, gardening, or just going for a walk.

D. Engage in hobbies: Hobbies and activities that you enjoy, such as painting, cooking, or playing a musical instrument, can provide a sense of accomplishment and help take your mind off of stressors.

E. Seek social support: Talking to friends and family, or joining a support group, can help reduce stress and improve your overall sense of well-being.

F. Get enough sleep: Lack of sleep can increase stress, so it's important to ensure you're getting enough rest.

G. Eat a healthy diet: A well-balanced diet can help you feel better physically, which can, in turn, help reduce stress.

H. Take breaks and engage in leisure activities: Make time for leisure activities and hobbies that you find enjoyable and relaxing.

I. Seek professional help: If your stress is severe or persistent, consider seeking help from a mental health professional.

Here are a few steps you can take:

a. Talk to your primary care doctor: Your doctor can help identify any underlying health issues contributing to our stress and recommend treatment options.

b. Consider seeing a mental health professional: Mental health professionals, such as therapists, psychologists, or psychiatrists, are trained to help people manage stress and other mental health concerns.

They can work with you to identify the causes of your stress and develop strategies for coping with it.

c. Research treatment options: There are many different types of treatment available for stress, including therapy, medication, and lifestyle changes. Research your options to find what might work best for you.

d. Reach out to support groups: Support groups can provide a sense of community and a safe space to share your feelings and experiences with others going through similar challenges.

e. Take care of yourself: In the meantime, make sure to take care of yourself by getting enough sleep, eating a healthy diet, and engaging in stress-reducing activities.

f. Ask for help: Don't be afraid to ask friends, family, or your primary care doctor for help finding a mental health professional or treatment program.

Remember, seeking help is a sign of strength, not weakness. It takes courage to admit that you need assistance, and seeking treatment can be an essential step toward improving your well-being.

Appendix

Tools for the Patient and Love-ones

In the following, when I say doctor, it also may mean a nurse who will meet with you. Talking to a nurse is acceptable; go with all of their suggestions. Nurses usually have more time to give you.

Support Groups

Cancer support groups are meetings that allow people with cancer to share their experiences and emotions with others in similar situations.

Below are a few of the many support groups. You may also use the search engine on the American Society of Clinical Oncology to search for more groups, ask your doctor or hospital, or use your favorite internet search engine.

Groups

American Society of Clinical Oncology (http://www.asco.org/) offers cancer patients and their families doctor-approved information; you can search for general cancer or cancer-specific support groups.

American Cancer Society (http://www.cancer.org/treatment.html) has the Cancer Survivors Network to help cancer survivors, families, and friends find and communicate with others who share their interests and experiences.

The Cancer Support Community (http://www.cancersupportcommunity. org/) is an international non-profit offering personalized services and education to support cancer patients.

Susan G. Komen for the Cure (http://ww5.komen.org/) is a non-profit organization created for breast cancer research and awareness.

CanCare (http://cancare.org/) is an online support network for cancer survivors and their families. This support comes from trained volunteers who have experienced and survived a cancer diagnosis or have been a caregiver to someone with cancer.

LIVESTRONG
(http://www.livestrong.com/) **is a global cancer support and research organization. They provide support and resources to all people affected by cancer.**

Imerman Angels
(http://imermanangels.org/) were created on the belief that no one should have to fight cancer alone and provides 1-on-1 cancer support by pairing those diagnosed with cancer with 'Mentor Angels' (survivors) who have survived the same kind of cancer.

4th Angel (http://www.4thangel.org/) provides free, one-on-one, confidential telephone support for cancer patients and their caregivers.

Inspire (http://www.inspire.com/) features groups for people with cancer and their caregivers. Once you join a group, you can post questions and comments on discussion boards and connect with other group members.

Know cancer (http://www.knowcancer.com/) is dedicated to connecting, educating, and empowering all people affected by cancer.

Smart Patients (http://www.smartpatients.com/) is an online community where patients and families affected by various illnesses can learn from each other about treatments, challenges, and how it all fits into the context of their experience.

Need a Ride to Treatment?

The American Cancer Society runs a free transportation service, a curbside-to-curbside, for patients to and from cancer-related treatments. Trained volunteers donate their time and vehicles to take you to and from treatment.

The cancer patient must have no means of transportation or cannot drive themselves.

The American Cancer Society transportation program is called "Road to Recovery." For more information, visit www.cancer.org/drive, contact your local American Cancer Society office, or call 1-899-227-2345.

Prepare for Doctor's Meeting

Make a written list of your questions. If you have a written list, you will get greater attention from your doctor. Keep a notepad or computer in one place to add to the list over time. It is best always to write everything down.

Bring a trusted person with you. You need a second set of ears. You are under stress, which reduces your listening abilities. They also might think of additional follow-up questions for the doctor.

Write down the doctor's answers and anything else relevant. Stress reduces your mental capacity to remember essential items.

Ask for printed information about your cancer and your treatment. Please ensure the doctor goes over the material, do not let the doctor hand it to you and then leave.

Find how and who to contact in an emergency.

Questions for your Doctor

This list is a good starting place; please add your questions.

Who is my principal doctor? The person I go to get any answers I need.

Which doctor will be prescribing me the pain medication?

How do I reach you, not just during business hours?

What is the stage of my cancer?

What are the risks of my treatment?

What type of treatment do you suggest?

What are the other options for treatment?

How long will treatment last?

Will I be able to drive to and from treatment?

What kind of cancer do I have?

How and how long before we know if the treatment is working?

How often do you treat this type of cancer?

Can you cure this cancer?

What are the possible side effects of this treatment?

What side-effects or problems should immediately tell you?

What should I expect at the end of treatment?

What should I do to get ready for treatment?

Is there a clinical trial that would help me?

Pain

I quit using pain meds (pain medication) mid-way through chemo/radiation treatment, except when I went to bed. I do not suggest that you stop your pain meds. My meds interfered with my thought process, preventing me from being on top of what was happening. The meds did not make the pain disappear; they made me a little high.

I strongly suggest you talk to only one doctor about your pain. Having multiple doctors prescribe pain meds could have disastrous effects. Have only one doctor prescribe pain meds to you.

Most people can find an excellent solution to their pain if they keep their doctor informed of the type of pain, the severity of the pain, and when it hurts.

Types of pain: Sharp, dull, stabbing, flashing, shooting, stinging, shock-like, tingling, numb, aching, cramping, pulling, pressing, pinching, crushing, cold, or burning. Use these terms to describe your pain to your doctor.

The severity of pain is rated 1 to 10. 1 being little pain. 10 being the worse pain possible.

When it hurts, does it start after something, at what time of day, how long does it hurt, and what makes it feel better?

Food

Diet is critical to your treatment. Try to eat as healthy as possible; find some things that you enjoy but are also healthy. Talk to your doctor for suggestions; your therapy may require special meals.

In my case of throat cancer, eating was not an option; I drank all of my meals (I don't mean booze).

You must not lose weight, even if you are overweight. Fat is used by your body for energy to rebuild the cells in your body. The cells cannot make you well if there is no fat. Be sure to talk to your doctor about your diet and your weight. The nurse should weigh you every time you come in for treatment.

Every time the nurse weights you, ask if your weight has gone up or down and is it okay. Your nurse will have to look up your previous weightings and make sure the nurse looks them up.

Over-the-Counter drugs

Talk to your doctor before you take any over-the-counter drugs, vitamins, minerals, herbs, or dietary supplements. I mean ANY THING! People mistakenly think that just because something is sold over the counter, it is safe to use in any situation.

No exceptions; talk to your doctor about anything you take.

Side Effects of Treatment

Expect to find some side effects, no matter what type of therapy you choose for your treatment.

Before starting treatment, an intern took a half-hour to tell me all the possible side effects. The list was so severe that I decided to drive home so that I would not have the chemo plus radiation treatment; I would have the surgery even though it was impossible because my cancer had spread so much. I eventually cooled down and went with the recommended therapy.

The list of side effects can be very long. The list is not known what will happen, but some of the items on the list might happen. In situations like yours, you must ask your doctor what to expect.

What to do, When Cancer Comes Back?

I know the pain of being told you are cured and then discovering that the cancer is back. In some respects, the second time around is worse.

When cancer comes back, it is called recurrence or recurrent cancer. My cancer had never truly gone away, so technically, it was not recurrent, just stubborn.

Sometimes new cancer develops not related to primary cancer. The second cancer is called a "second primary cancer."

When your disease returns or you get a second disease, you may become less hopeful than ever. Now is the time to talk about how you feel to your loved ones, support group, or doctor.

Today cancer is considered a chronic illness; it can come back a second and third time. The disease becomes an ongoing (chronic) illness. It may never go away.

When cancer comes back, it does not mean that you will die. It would help if you talked to your doctor about treatment, the chance of recovery, and your fears.

A Place to Stay

The American Cancer Society has a program called "Hope Lodge." Call them at (800) 227-2345 to see if it is available in your area.

The program provides a free home away from home for cancer patients and their caregivers when they travel far from home to get treatment. If not available in your area, there is the "Hotel Partners Program." This program gives patients and their caregivers a reduced rate or a complimentary stay in hotels close to their treatment.

Finances

We have all seen articles where a family loses all their money to hospital costs. It may take a little work searching, but there are many ways to pay for treatment.

Medical insurance is your first line of defense; if you have it, talk to your insurance agent to find out what they will cover. The hospital often has a department that will speak to your insurance company for you.

Your hospital should have someone to assist you in finding ways to pay for your treatment.

Most hospitals are required by law to assist you or eliminate payments for treatment. Ask your doctor or nurse who to talk to if that department has not contacted you. The doctor or nurse cannot help with your finances but can direct you to someone that can help you.

Pharmaceutical manufacturers also have programs to help you pay for their drugs. Find out which drug you will get (except for surgery) and the manufacturer. If you need help paying for their drug, they will help you.

American Cancer Society can help you with finances.

Contact the American Cancer Society at:
Call: 1-800-813-HOPE (1-800-813-4673)
Visit: www.cancercare.org
email: info@cancercare.org

Alternative Therapy (non-Western Medicine)

Many hospitals offer some forms of alternative treatment while you are receiving your main form of Therapy (chemo, radiation, surgery, etc.).

I am not a medical doctor, but I know this as an absolute fact; you will die if you use only alternative medicine to treat your cancer.

Steve Jobs (co-founder of Apple) would tell you the same thing if he was alive today. Steve told a friend when his friend got same cancer as him, "go for western medicine from the start, do not do what I did."

Some alternative medicines can help you when used in conjunction with western medicine.

Meditation and yoga can help reduce your stress level.

Stress can lower your white cell count. Your white cells fight infections.

Talk to your doctor about what else can be done to get you on the road to recovery.

Is Cancer Contagious?

No.

About the Author (Geoffrey L. Lefavi)

I was a successful computer consultant working with multinational companies.

Jeff's other non-fiction books:
"Stop Procrastination," "10 Steps to a Better Brain", and "The Mueller Report, Volume I & II."

Jeff has written science-fictions books:
"Rubix – Saving Humanity," "Albert – Saving Humanity," and "Matthew – Saving Humanity.

More books to come.

###

Thank you for reading my book. If you enjoyed it, please take a moment to leave a review at your favorite retailer.

I am not a medical doctor; I will not respond to medical questions.

If you have any comments, questions or concerns, please email me at:
BooksByJeff@yahoo.com

Thank you,
Jeff

The Pathway

15 Months - no valid diagnosis.

3 Months - to start treatment.

8 Months - to find out Chemo & Radiation did not work.

2 Years - new drug treatment with no visible cancer.

2 Years later – off of the drug, hopefully forever.

I did not give the drug name because I feared people would think this new miracle drug would save them.

There are many types of cancers and many types of drugs.

You will find your miracle by never giving up.

A Note to Family and Friends of Cancer Patients

You are under intense stress. Your stress is detrimental to your family members or cancer patient.

Alcohol does not cure stress. There is a long list of ways to reduce your stress.

Your cancer patient is stressed and needs someone to be there.

People under stress can make bad decisions and cause increased stress for cancer patients.

Be understanding of outbursts from the patient.

It would help if you were the patient's second eyes and ears. Write everything down. Keep track of the patient's diet, pain, and mental acuity. Everything the nurse or doctor says you need to write down. Keep your notes well organized.

Try some of these things to reduce stress and see if the patient will do them with you. You do not need to do them all; just a few can be very helpful.

1. **Meditation**

The goal of meditation is to quiet the mind and relax thoughts. It involves concentrating on a simple image or sound while in a comfortable place away from distractions.

2. **Massage**

A massage may slow down the heart and relax the body. Rather than causing drowsiness, a massage increases alertness and feels excellent.

3. **Maintaining Healthy Habits**

People who deal with stress will resort to unhealthy habits, including high-fat and high-salt diets, tobacco use, alcohol abuse, and a sedentary lifestyle.

4. **Getting regular Aerobic Exercise**

A brisk walk can reduce the level of stress hormones in your blood. At least 30 minutes a day (or two 15-minute sessions) is best, but even three times a week offers benefits.

5. **Dance**

Dancing is a great aerobic exercise; it helps you build a social network and does not seem like exercise. Dancing allows you to listen to music, exercise physically, and expand your social network.

6. **Listening to Music**

Listening to music will decrease anxiety levels. Music lowers your blood pressure and heart rate, changes plasma stress hormone levels, affects your respiration, reduces muscle tension, increases endorphin levels, and boosts your immune system.

7. **More Music, Less TV**

As stated above, listening to music will reduce your stress. Not watching television will reduce your stress. Many people leave the television on, even not watching the program. We have found that having the TV on as background noise increases your stress levels.

8. **Do Yoga**

Some do yoga for the stretching benefits, some for the stretching & cardiovascular benefits, and others because it relaxes them.

9. **Call Friends**

Talking to your friends about your problems helps you relieve anxiety (stress).

10. **Read Food Labels**

Your mind and body are firmly attached; they affect each other. You must keep your body in good condition to keep your mind in shape, and vice versa.

11. **Aromatherapy**

Aromatherapy is over-hyped these days, making many extraordinary claims. It may not help all people. But it can help some people relax, thereby avoiding and reducing stress. Find the scent that enables you to relax and use it.

12. **Get a Dog**

Man's best friend is a way to a healthier life. They are always happy to see you come home and ready to play anytime. Studies have found that just petting a dog lowers your blood pressure. A pet can be an excellent means of reducing stress.

13. **Sleep**

Get seven to eight hours of deep sleep per night. To get a night of proper deep sleep, take a hot shower or bath just before bed. Go to bed at the same time each night; you will fall asleep faster and more rested sleep.

14. **Drink Tea**

Studies have shown that tea: lowers the risk of heart attack, reduces "bad" cholesterol, fights cancer, reduces inflammation in arthritis patients, and reduces stress. Tea contains the amino acid L-Theanine, which has been shown to promote relaxation.

15. **Medication**

Stress-reducing medication ordered by your physician is usually your last resort, but if you need it, YOU NEED IT. Let your physician be your guide.

16. **Get Some Sun**

You need about ten minutes of direct sunlight every day for your body to make enough vitamin "D" required by your body, but talk to your doctor first).

17. **Nature Photo**

Place a photo of a pastoral sight on your nightstand so you can gaze at it when you open your eyes. Studies have shown that viewing images of nature reduces blood pressure and muscle tension within five minutes.

www.ingramcontent.com/pod-product-compliance
Lightning Source LLC
Chambersburg PA
CBHW030639220526
45463CB00004B/1573